MOSQUITO

Richard Swift is a co-editor of the *New Internationalist* magazine.

Trigger Issues
One small item – one giant impact

Other titles:
Kalashnikov
Diamonds

MOSQUITO

Richard Swift

NEW INTERNATIONALIST

595·772
(77415)

Trigger Issues: Mosquito
First published in the UK in 2006 by
New Internationalist™ Publications Ltd
55 Rectory Road
Oxford OX4 1BW, UK
www.newint.org
New Internationalist is a registered trade mark.

Cover: Mosquito. Will Crocker/The Image Bank

Series editor: Troth Wells
Design by New Internationalist Publications Ltd.

 Printed on recycled paper by T J International, Cornwall, UK
who hold environmental accreditation ISO 14001.

British Library Cataloguing-in-Publication Data.
A catalogue record for this book is available from the British Library.

Library of Congress Cataloguing-in-Publication Data.
A catalogue for this book is available from the Library of Congress.

ISBN 10: 1-904456-31-6
ISBN 13: 978-1904456-315

Contents

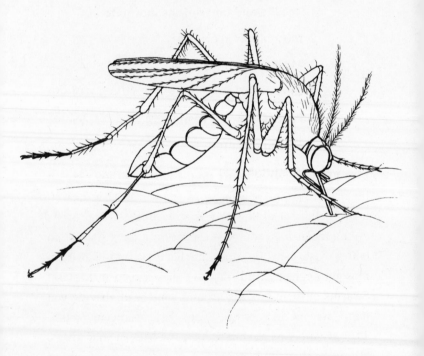

1

The life and times of the mosquito

'The good Lord didn't create anything without a purpose, but mosquitoes come close.'

Mosquitoes – who needs them? Not like they play an important role in the ecosystem as a whole. They aren't a major pollinator of flowers like other insects. They aren't even a major food source – except for a few bats and an odd grayish fish (the Mosquito Fish) that specializes in mosquito cuisine. And man are they a pain in the ass! Swarms of them buzzing around your head, driving you nuts. They are in your eyes, your ears, even your mouth. They are nibbling at your ankles, the back of your knees. Or maybe that single mozzie keeping you awake for hour after hour as it dive bombs you in your bed. Giving you those itchy bites. Ruining the picnic, the view, the garden.

When the salt marsh mosquito (*aedes taeniorhynchus*) swarms in the mangroves of the Florida Everglades in June some claim they block out the sun. On the 'mosquito flyway' that comes out of the Everglades and out over Key Island on the Florida Gulf Coast the high-pitched hum of their beating wings fills the air. A fancy resort (the Keewaydin Club) stands deserted on the 2-mile long Key. According to Gene Lemire of the local District authority: 'We have mosquitoes so bad that in 1989, they were killing cows. The cows were inhaling so many mosquitoes they were choking, suffocating.'[1] Further north there are even stories in the Canadian northwoods about camp sites that have been found with the bodies of campers completely covered in feasting flies. But that's all hearsay.

Bad neighbors

Mosquitoes (like humans?) are bad species neighbors. For all the obvious reasons but also because mosquitoes have a dirty little secret. They carry disease around with them. Lots of disease: pathogens – the infectious agents, such as bacteria or viruses. Often quite deadly or at least debilitating. They take them from one horse to another.

From one bird to another. From one monkey to another. From one person to another. But they can also carry them across species. Carrying them from individual-to-individual makes the mosquito a 'vector', from species-to-species makes them a 'bridge vector'. In this age of global worry about pandemics of flu and runaway viruses the old mozzie is taking center stage.

But we'd better get used to the mosquito because they are a major evolutionary success story and despite the efforts of humans, they aren't going away any time soon. Humankind (or at least those 'representatives' that get to decide for us) has brought the full weight of industrial science to eradicate the pest and the results have been partial at best. An arsenal of chemical and pharmaceutical weaponry has been deployed. While hundreds of thousands of lives have been saved by the use of the chemical DDT and other measures, the 1950s and 1960s' military language of eradication and liquidation has proved wildly optimistic. The conquest of the winged wonder is in a way a metaphor for the whole 'domination of nature' and has had similar results. The mosquito, like nature, continues to bite back.

With a bit of variation the life cycle of a mosquito such as the common domestic mosquito of temperate climes

LIFE-CYCLE

It's pretty risky being a mosquito. Your mother ends up leaving you in some stagnant water... a pond or clogged gutter.

You get left with a few hundred of your brothers and sisters in an egg raft. Your egg may be destroyed before it even hatches. Or you do get to hatch and reach the stage of being a larva or even a pupa but there is just not enough to eat.

Then right away they are out to get you. Whether it is mosquito fish wanting to make a meal of you or a scary water strider trying to grab you. As you develop you become more appetizing to birds, frogs, snakes and spiders.

Say you become a *pupa*. Your troubles have only started. Your little mosquito body is starting to take shape and you need to start breathing air. You develop two breathing tubes that you stick above the water for some air. Now you are moving on to the *imago* stage and you can leave your *pupae* cuticle behind. If you are able to stay out of harm's way until your cuticle splits open things start to move along pretty dramatically. You lose the ability to swim but you gain a set of wings and you can take off. You've got half an hour to get out of the water and find a safe refuge where your soft body can harden into a young mosquito. This usually takes a day or two. Now you are ready to boogey!

But you certainly aren't out of the metaphorical hot water. There are still predators who want to vacuum you up including that most deadly of mosquito serial killers: the bat. These guys can grab you at night when you are flying along and think that you can't even be seen. It's almost as if they had radar.

Say you feel like a night out and decide as a young female that you should head down to the swarm that the guys have put together to attract you. They can tell it's a girl by the beating of your wings and, man, are they glad to see you! You cut one out of the herd and before long there is a little abdominal action and you are in the family way. Your eggs are fertilized and you have some new needs. Not chocolate but a bit of blood is what you crave.

You need to find a mammal to provide the blood for those eggs. Here you have to be careful. Best to sneak in unnoticed, and use your two stylets to break the surface of the skin. If you can get your proboscis into a blood vessel you are home free. You can use one tube of your proboscis to suck up the red stuff while you stick some of your saliva from the other tube to prevent their blood from clotting. This keeps the flow nice and steady and it's not really your concern what's in the saliva you leave behind.

It takes about two minutes to fill up. You find a bit of surface to settle on and let the food digest. But watch out! The nutrients in a blood meal are attractive to predators. Does it never stop?

Then it's off to find some stagnant water where you can download those eggs. That's a relief. Only problem is that when you finish doing that your life is pretty much over. It's all taken about three weeks. Got to ask yourself – was it worth it? ◆

From Bobbie Kalman, *The Life Cycle of a Mosquito* (Crabtree Publishing Company, 2004).

– the *Culex pipiens* – is pretty much like that described in the box. Some mosquitoes however can live for five or six months. Some go into hibernation. Some species try to guard their egg rafts. One type, the *Anopheles salbaii*, an African desert dweller, doesn't need a blood meal to reproduce.

The eggs of some can survive in desert or arctic conditions for very long periods, in the case of one Sahara mosquito through decades of drought before a rainfall finally completes fertilization. And some (the most dangerous) mosquitoes take a blood meal more than once. Others are very particular where they take their blood from, such as a Canadian type which will bite only Loons (not mad people, but the Canadian national bird, an aquatic fowl). Yet others will bite across species and pass on infection say from monkeys or birds to people. Remember, the older the mosquito, the more likely they have some kind of nasty surprise with their bite.

Champion of adaptation

Given the precariousness of their lives it seems a wonder the mosquito is still with us. After all, almost 50 per cent never make it through their first day. But the pesky critters are evolutionary survivors *par excellence*. They

MOSQUITO DEFINED

In English, the word *Mosquito* (Spanish, *little fly*) dates back to 1583; the word was adopted to replace the term 'biting flies' to prevent confusion with the house fly. It is derived from the word *musca* and is related to the Italian *moschetta* and the French *moustique*. Mosquitoes are arthropods, an insect classification which constitutes over 90 per cent of the animal kingdom.

Why do they bite?

Mosquitoes belong to a group of insects that require blood to develop fertile eggs. Males do not lay eggs, thus, male mosquitoes do not bite. The females are the egg producers and 'host-seek' for a blood meal.

Both male and female feed on plant nectar, fruit juices and liquids that ooze from plants. The sugar is burned as fuel for flight. Blood is reserved for egg production and is imbibed less frequently.

Why are some people more attractive to mosquitoes then others?

Scientists are still investigating the complexities involved with mosquito host acceptance and rejection. Some people are highly attractive and others are rarely bothered. Mosquitoes have specific requirements to satisfy and process many different factors before they feed. ◆

Wikipedia http://en.wikipedia.org

have been around since the time of the dinosaurs and witnessed a lot of other species come and go. They survive, indeed prosper, from Himalayan mountain slopes up to 11,000 feet to below sea level in Baja California. The aggressive *Aedes communis* swarms north of the Arctic Circle literally eating the poor caribou alive. While down in Eritrea's Danakil Depression, one of the hottest places on earth, the mosquito has also learned to get by. So hot or cold, high or low, dry or wet (although wet is preferable) mozzies find a way.

The mosquito is a member of the family *Culicidae*. Altogether there are between 2,500 and 3,000 different types of mosquito with an estimated global population of 100 trillion (although God knows how anyone can really tell). They are also implicated as the greatest killers of humans. Between one and three million die of malaria alone every year and this says nothing about a range of other mosquito-borne diseases – West Nile virus, yellow fever, dengue, and various forms of encephalitis. The mosquito bite itself, while certainly annoying, is not what spreads the disease. But certain types of mosquitoes act as what are called 'disease vectors' carrying 'pathogens' (infectious agents) including viruses they pick up from one mammal to infect another.

Mozzie types

There are three main genus of mosquito – *Anopheles*, the *Culex* and the *Aedes*. The main culprit in the transmission of malaria is *Anopheles*, a type of warm weather mosquito. Of the 400 or so mosquito species of genus *Anopheles* about 60 transmit the *plasmodium* parasites that cause malaria. Species in the *Anopheles gambaie* are the main spreaders of malaria in Africa where the human toll amongst children results in about 90 per cent of malaria cases and deaths.

The *Culex* is the most common mosquito in the Northern hemisphere and the least likely to carry dangerous pathogens although it can carry viral encephalitis and filariasis (also known as elephantiasis) in tropical and sub-tropical regions. Recently it was discovered that certain types of the *Culex* are also a vector for West Nile virus.

The genus *Aedes* during its short life span can carry yellow fever, dengue and also encephalitis. Some of the *Aedes* are known as 'house mosquitoes' because of their tendency to breed in domestic locales in rain/water barrels, birdbaths, buckets and so on. Their short life and local range make it possible to cut down on their population by eliminating all domestic breeding habitats. This is one of the ways health authorities have been able to get on top of the peril of yellow fever. Other *Aedes* are the salt marsh variety known for their fierce swarming that can drive various mammals (including us) almost mad with the desire to escape. They are more easily subjected to aerial spraying because of their location and tendency towards large-scale swarming.

Mosquito-borne diseases

It was only in the last couple of decades of the 19th century that suspicions were finally confirmed that mosquitoes were a major carrier of a number of dangerous diseases. While this ended centuries of blind panic in the face of mysterious epidemics and plagues, it started a mortal combat between people and the winged tormentors. The outcome is still undecided. The following are the main diseases that we now recognize are spread by mosquito bite.

Malaria

Malaria, derived from *mal aria* (Italian for 'bad air') and formerly called 'ague' or 'marsh fever' in English, was originally thought to be produced by 'miasma' or poisoned air. According to the World Health Organization, more than 3 billion people (roughly half the world's population) live under the threat of malaria. Each year, the disease causes about 350-500 million infections in humans and kills about 1.3 million – mostly children. It remains the deadliest disease for which the mosquito acts as a vector. It is the most common of tropical diseases, killing mainly the already weakened or vulnerable (by disease, age or malnutrition) or the very young who have no immunity built up. Sub-Saharan Africa is home to some 90 per cent of the world's malaria cases and deaths.

Once inside the body the malaria parasite multiplies in the liver and red blood cells. Severe cases suffer alternately from frigid chills that can lead to violent shakes, and bouts of high fever that can reach 106° Fahrenheit. The victim's red blood cells are made sticky by the parasite clogging their vascular system and starving the brain and other vital organs of oxygen. For the dying the sequence is lethargy, delirium and finally coma. Some historians estimate that during the Second World War US forces in the Pacific lost more troops to malaria than to the Japanese.

Yellow fever
This causes fever, jaundice and hemorrhages that eventually kill a great number of those who contract it. Yellow fever (or Yellow Jack as it used to be called) can result in the most terrible of deaths involving

MOSQUITOES – THE NUMBERS

The average female mosquito's wings beat between 250 to 500 times a second.

A mosquito can hit a top speed of about 3 miles an hour.

Mosquitoes fly about 150 miles in their lifetime.

Most mosquitoes live within one mile of where they have been hatched. A few species can range up to 20 miles.

A female mosquito usually lives from 3 to 100 days. A male from 10 to 20 days.

A female may lay 1,000 to 3,000 eggs over the course of its lifetime.

Biting activity can increase up to 500 times with a full moon.

The female mosquito can suck up to three times its body weight in blood.

20 per cent of people receive 80 per cent of bites from infected mosquitoes.

MALARIA – THE NUMBERS

There are between 300,000 and 500,000 new cases of clinical malaria every year.

The global death toll from malaria and malaria-related diseases is over 1 million people each year.

Depending where they live, people in Africa can receive anywhere between one to 1,000 infective mosquito bites per year. By contrast the average in Latin America or Southeast Asia is one infective bite most years.

Africa is home to around 90 per cent of the world's malaria cases and related deaths. In Kenya 11 per cent of schooldays are lost every year because of the disease.

Children (mostly African) can have as many as 5 different strains of malaria in them at once.

The disease costs Africa between $3 and $12 billion a year but could be controlled for much less. ◆

www.mosquitozapper.com/facts; 'Combating Malaria', Anne Platt McGinn, *State of the World's Children Report 2003*, UNICEF.

uncontrollable bleeding and vomiting. In the past, it was feared for its intensity and the rapidity with which it spread. The so-called 'ghost ships' like the famous *Flying Dutchman* found abandoned, floating lifeless in the ocean, were probably a consequence of yellow fever.

In her book *Yellow Fever and the South*, Margaret Holmes quotes a letter from a man who watched his daughter die: 'Jaundice was marked, the skin being a bright yellow hue; tongue and lips dark, cracked and blood oozing from the mouth and nose... to me the most terrifying feature was the black vomit which I never before witnessed. By Tuesday it was black as ink and would be ejected with terrific force.'[2] The yellow fever virus can still be found in wild primates in Africa and the Americas. It is much less of a threat than it used to be (there are effective vaccines for those who can afford them); however it remains a problem particularly in relatively remote jungle areas.

Dengue

Dengue is known as 'break-bone fever' because of the acute skeletal pain associated with the disease. There are four distinct types of dengue fever (DF), but only one dengue hemorrhagic fever (DHF – a combination of two types of dengue) is likely to be fatal. The disease occurs at various spots throughout the Global South. In 1970 dengue was found in nine countries, while today it is in 60. As with yellow fever, dengue is spread by *Aedes aegypti*. By 2005 the disease had a global distribution comparable to that of malaria with an estimated 2.5 billion people living in risk areas. Each year, tens of millions of cases of DF occur and depending on the year up to hundreds of thousands of cases of DHF. The case-fatality rate of DHF in most countries is about five per cent. But with proper treatment this could be reduced to below one per cent. It is mostly the young who die.

Encephalitis

This is caused by the encephalitis virus, an 'arbovirus'. Arbovirus is short for **ar**thropod-**bo**rne **virus**. There are several types, including the St Louis (SLE), Western Equine (WEE) and Eastern Equine (EEE) encephalitis. The last two are viral diseases transmitted to horses and humans by mosquitoes; but the virus that causes EEE cannot be passed from horses to humans. Once contracted, the virus can result in an inflammation of the brain and the membrane that surrounds it. This can lead to mild outcomes such as flu-like symptoms, but can be

MOSQUITO

....crawling into my head, mosquito, mosquito red pieces,
diseases, floating in the greases, but they smile instead

sting of the suckerfly
in the dead of the night
ride on the wings of a dragonfly
sleep by the candlelight
sucking the gutter dry
taking flight
now they dance on the open eye
pushing the needle to the tiny bite

watching the circling sun, mosquito, mosquito run
vision of a killing gun
they sing with the voices of the angels son

river is flowing
the bloody wind is blowing
the reaper they are sowing
and i don't believe that they are going

crawling into my eye, mosquito, mosquito fly
falling from the scientist slide
eating at the walls from behind they hide...

Psychotic Waltz, US progressive metal band

lethal in some cases. EEE is the most serious with older victims dying of their infection while the young enter a semi-comatose state that gives EEE its more popular designation as 'sleeping sickness'. EEE often has 'swamp mosquitoes' (*Culiseta melanura*) as its main vector. These are particularly active in wet conditions and feed mostly on birds that become the reservoir of EEE. The birds are then bitten by other mozzies that also bite humans. Such mosquitoes are known as 'bridge vectors' as they transfer pathogens from one species to another.

West Nile virus

This affects mainly birds but can be found in a number of mammals including humans and horses. It is transmitted by varieties of the *Culex* mosquito and was first discovered in Uganda just before the Second World War. It has almost no effect on 80 per cent of the people who contract it but does cause a mild fever in a minority. An even smaller minority of mostly older victims get quite sick with symptoms of fever, nausea and even paralysis. Death occurs in a small minority of cases. No effective treatment is known. The geographic spread of West Nile virus has increased dramatically because of the migratory habits of bird hosts and the very common mosquito vectors that also act as bridge vectors between birds and mammals. In 1999, after a few fatal cases in New York City, the mayor had the whole city doused with insecticide.

Filariasis

This is spread by the *filaria* worm. It can cause extreme disfigurement and is commonly known as elephantiasis. This is one of the diseases with the highest level of social stigma attached to it (like leprosy) because of the dramatic disfigurements that frequently accompany it: everything from genitals to limbs can be swollen almost out of recognition. Although the disease is seldom fatal, secondary infections following surgical intervention may cause death. It was with filariasis that a British doctor, Patrick Manson, first suggested a link to the mosquito. Manson worked in Taiwan in the 1870s where he saw hundreds of cases and did initial research that identified the mosquito as the vector bearing the filaria worm. Today full-blown elephantiasis is rare due to overall improvements in health, mosquito control programs and the use of the drug Ivermectin to control infection before it gets out of hand.

Another type of filarial infection which also occurs in the tropics is 'river blindness' (*Onchocerciasis*) that literally renders those affected sightless if not properly treated.

2 Mosquitoes in history

'When did you start your tricks, Monsieur?'

FROM DH LAWRENCE, *THE MOSQUITO*

It wasn't until the 1890s that the mosquito was identified as a source of sickness. Before that, most disease was either attributed to certain types of people (those of color and from strange parts) or to foul air and water. But since that time historians have identified the likely effect of mosquito-borne diseases on earlier epochs of human history.

The defeat of many invading armies, and deaths of Popes and Emperors, can be seen as at least partially influenced by the lowly mosquito. In his play *Julius Caesar* Shakespeare wrote:

He had the fever when he was in Spain
And when the fit was on him, I did mark
How he did shake.

In Italy it became a commonplace that invaders and strangers were subject to feverish illnesses when they spent too much time in central regions. The poet Godfrey of Viterbo caught the flavor of this in 1167 when he penned, 'When unable to defend herself by the sword, Rome could defend herself by means of the fever.' The Pontin Marshes south of Rome were one source of malarial infection carried to the City by its winged avengers. Visigoths and Huns were just some of the 'barbarian hordes' that fell foul of disease. Centuries later, in the Middle Ages, French and German Popes died of malaria. In their retreat up the Italian peninsula during World War Two the German Army broke dikes and re-flooded the Pontin Marshes to create an epidemic of malaria amongst the advancing allied troops – but of course it killed many Italians too (see box).

The Roman case sets a pattern whereby a local population has developed a relative immunity while outsiders are devastated by mosquito-borne diseases like malaria and yellow fever. Some historians now feel it is likely that Alexander the Great died from malaria in 323 BCE and that the armies of Genghis Khan were so

STING IN THE TAIL

In Italy, malaria was not just a medical problem, but a social and regional issue too. Politics was transformed by the anti-malarial campaigns. It was decided to give quinine to all people in certain regions. The strategy was successful: deaths fell by some 80 per cent in the first decade of the 20th century. Mussolini's policies in the 1920s and 1930s instituted mass draining of the marshes – but involved forced population removals. The cleansing of Italy was also ethnic as 'carefully selected' Italians were chosen to inhabit the gleaming new towns of the former marshlands around Rome. As war swept through the drained lands in the 1940s, the disease returned.

In 'the only known example of biological warfare in 20th-century Europe', the retreating Nazi armies in 1943-44 deliberately caused a huge malaria epidemic in Lazio. They flooded the plains causing maximum damage to the local population – an example of 'total war' waged on civilians. Ironically it was the jewel in Mussolini's crown – the new city of Littoria (now Latina) – which suffered the worst damage at the hands of his own allies. Fifty-five thousand cases of malaria were recorded in the province of Littoria in 1944. ◆

From *John Foot*'s review of *The Conquest of Malaria in Italy, 1900-1962* by Frank M Snowden (Yale, 2006), *The Guardian* 8 April 2006.

devastated by the disease that they were prevented from invading Europe.

The history of colonialism and imperialism is marked by the wily mosquito. In the Americas the indigenous people refer to the death of millions through exposure to such European diseases as measles, smallpox, typhus and cholera as 'a holocaust'. Indeed it was. But the white colonialists and slavers were to suffer a similar fate in their exposure to mosquito-borne diseases that Africans had gained at least partial immunity to. Such diseases were carried in slave-ships to the Americas as the colonial enterprise sought to replace the devastated indigenous population with African slave labor. Mozzies got aboard the slave ships (and moved through their life cycle in the course of the voyage likely laying eggs in drinking water containers). They bit the slaves (already infected and with a degree of immunity) and also the crew who lacked immunity and succumbed. This process was seen as one reason slaves were able to seize the ship *Amistad* in mid-ocean. But mostly the slavers brought their cargo into port, inadvertently helping establish the mosquito population, malaria and yellow fever in the Americas.

Such diseases particularly affected European colonial armies in the New World. When the French tried to retake Haiti in 1802 after its Black Jacobin revolt they fell foul not only of stiff resistance from the former slaves but also had their modern army of 29,000 devastated by disease so that only 6,000 survived. Although the French killed over 150,000 Haitians, they were eventually driven out.

But it was in Africa itself that the colonists really suffered. In the UK, the West African coast became known as 'the white man's graveyard' and as one popular little ditty had it:

Beware, beware the Bight of Benin
One comes out where fifty went in.[3]

Perhaps it should have been 'Bite' of Benin. First for explorers and then for the colonial enterprise as a whole the mosquito proved a deadly foe. Eventually white colonization was limited to a few cities, highland areas and strategically important mines and other sites in much of sub-Saharan Africa. Europeans suffered a similar if slightly less dramatic fate throughout Asia and the South Seas.

Race and mosquitoes

Whether explorers or troops, white men suffered most dramatically from mosquito-borne diseases. When slave ships landed in the Americas, their crews were often sick and the illness spread quickly in places such as the American South. Cities including Philadelphia, Memphis and New Orleans suffered from terrible waves of disease. No-one knew exactly where the malady came from but it became fixed in the public mind as associated with the tropics, travelers and people of color. According to Henry Rose Carter, chief medical officer for the state of Mississippi, yellow fever was 'imported by Negroes'. It was of course beyond the comprehension of the time that certain people (black or white) could develop immunity to such diseases while still carrying them in their blood.

The mixture of plague panic and racism often resulted in attacks on black people and strangers. Lynching and beatings were common. In one incident in Louisiana six Italian immigrants were blamed for fraternizing with black people and spreading yellow fever. They were lynched.

This view went beyond a populist no-nothingism to the center of scientific thinking. Ronald Ross, who won the Nobel Prize for establishing the mosquito as the source of malaria transmission, held to the conventional prejudice. He believed that malaria struck down 'not only the indigenous barbaric population but with greater certainty, the pioneers of civilization – the planter, the trader, the missionary, the soldier. It is therefore the principal and gigantic ally of Barbarism.' Colonial policy mirrored Ross's view with anti-malarial efforts aimed at creating safe and separate spaces for a cloistered colonial élite while the indigenous population was left to its own devices.

Africans took a more benign view of the sufferings of their colonial masters, enveloped by swarms of mozzies. A 19th-century African popular song catches the flavor:

The poor white man faint and weary
Come to sit under our tree
He has no mother to bring him milk
No wife to grind his corn
Let us pity the poor white man.[2]

The fact that the causes of malaria and other mosquito-borne diseases were unknown contributed to some quite strange theories of causation focusing on everything from 'earthly emanations', filth and poor air to immorality and bad character. During the French attempt to build the Panama Canal, as Spielman and D'Antonio point out in their book *Mosquito*[2]: 'One of the project engineers even came to believe that he could predict which of the newly-arrived workers would sicken and die, based solely on the expressions on their faces as they came ashore. Another engineer said that he would prove that only the immoral would die – by bringing his family to Panama. Not long after their arrival, his son, daughter and son-in-law were all dead of yellow fever. He would lose his wife before succumbing himself.'

The Panama Canal

When the French financier Ferdinand de Lesseps (1805-1894) took on construction of a shipping canal to link the Atlantic to the Pacific across the Isthmus of Panama in 1881 there were few doubters. After all, here was the main force behind the building of the Suez Canal and a towering figure in French finance and engineering. Investors flocked to put their money into what they were sure would be the lucrative realization of a centuries-old dream. No expense was spared and some of the finest housing compounds ever seen in the tropics were built for the workers. They were complete with lavish gardens where various water features – inadvertently – allowed mosquitoes ample breeding opportunities. Little provision was made for screening to keep out what were thought of as mere pests. Those who pointed out that the area was 'disease-ridden' were simply dismissed.

The toll was horrendous. The loss of life, individual fortunes, national prestige and personal reputations would take many decades to live down. The workers started dropping like flies from the first survey party. Thousands fell, including entire crews from some ships, from malaria and yellow fever. Where the disease came from no-one knew. It was most popularly seen as a kind of character flaw or punishment for immoral behavior.

In fact of course it was the handiwork of that pesky little mosquito. As 1884 drew to a close 1,200 men had died in that year alone and all attempts to keep the tragedy quiet and the investors in the game were proving futile. Coffins were piled up beside the train stations and on the docks. Altogether an estimated 30,000 succumbed including de Lesseps himself, who reportedly lapsed into a 'melancholic kind of senility'. The famous French engineer Eiffel was made to pay a huge fine for his role in the fiasco. The tiny mosquito had again stolen the show.

By the time of the next attempt to finish the work on the Canal things had changed. It was 1904 and pioneering doctors and scientists had begun to identify the mosquito as the source of malaria and yellow fever. The key player this time was US Army Surgeon-General William Crawford Gorgas (1854-1920) who had been one of a number of important figures in identifying and then combating mosquito infestation in Cuba during the American occupation of that country a couple of years before the Canal project (see below).

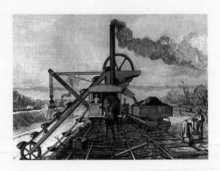

Gorgas had the job of keeping the US workforce healthy in Panama. It was a pretty tall order. Not only did he have to make inroads into the mosquito population and try to keep the workers and the insects separate, he had to do it while dealing with a skeptical project administration. His commanding officer Admiral John Walker thought that the connection between mosquitoes and disease was 'balderdash'. Walker and others did everything they could to frustrate the determined (some said heavy-handed) Gorgas' efforts to combat disease. Indeed some of his approaches were not that well thought-out – such as the attempt to vaccinate the workers by keeping a supply of recently infected mosquitoes to give them a mild case of yellow fever. More successful was his program of screening off those infected (and screening in general) and the use of oil and drainage to destroy mosquito breeding habitat in the immediate region. In the end Gorgas' strategies proved remarkably successful in virtually eradicating yellow fever and vastly reducing the incidence of the more persistent malaria. In the decade it took to finish the Canal only two per cent of the workforce was hospitalized at any one time. Under the French the total had been at least 30 per cent.

Mosquito unmasked

When the mosquito began to be recognized (quite painfully and reluctantly) as a disease vector things really started to heat up. The scientists and public health officials making this startling discovery had to convince the-powers-that-be that it wasn't damp air or moral failings that caused disease. The decades preceding and following the turn of the 20th century were exciting ones. The names of the key figures – Patrick Manson, Charles Laveran, Ronald Ross, the New Jersey chief epidemiologist John Smith,

James Carroll and William Gorgas of Panama Canal fame are all now part of the Pantheon of Public Health. Some, like the illustrious US military doctor Walter Reed (1851-1902) garnered the lion's share of the credit, while others such as the Cuban Carlos Juan Finlay (1833-1915) had his achievements marginalized because he wasn't of the right race or ethnicity. As early as 1865 Dr Finlay had sent a paper to the Academy of Sciences in Havana theorizing that a mosquito was the means by which yellow fever was transmitted (see box).

Havana at the end of the 19th century was buzzing with discovery and innovation. The US had occupied Cuba under the pretext of helping the Cubans gain their independence from Spain. However in a pattern to be established throughout Latin America and beyond, it proved quite difficult to get rid of the US military once it was embedded on your soil. But the heavy toll taken by tropical disease on US troops and other personnel, particularly from yellow fever and malaria, caused resources and research to be devoted to finding a solution. Some creative sleuthing inspired by Manson's work on yellow fever in Taiwan, Ross's on malaria in Calcutta and Finlay's locally began to identify mosquitoes as a source of the problem.

UNSUNG HERO

One of the earliest medical pioneers to identify the mosquito as a disease vector was Dr Carlos Finlay of Cuba. In 1865 Finlay published his suspicions that yellow fever was spread by mosquito bite. By 1880 he was experimenting with letting yellow fever-infected mosquitoes give controlled doses of the disease to the previously uninfected as a form of inoculation. His work was viewed with skepticism by a medical establishment convinced that 'filth' was the cause of most disease. His work was also sidelined because of his humble Cuban origins outside the mainstream of Euro-American medicine. But during the US occupation medical experts like Dr Walter Reed were exposed not only to the ravages of yellow fever but also to Finlay's work which gradually began to gain credibility. The 1900 Commission headed by Reed also did experiments and Reed eventually announced that 'our theory' of disease transmission had been proved. In his report Reed did not even bother to mention Finlay and his 20 years of experiments on mosquitoes and yellow fever. It was only in 1959, 39 years after Finlay's death, that the International Congress of Medical History granted him proper credit.

Since 1980 UNESCO has awarded the biennial Carlos J Finlay Prize to a person or a group working for an outstanding contribution to microbiology. ◆

Three doctors associated with the Reed Commission (see box p 37) – James Carroll, Aristedes Agramonte and Jesse Lazear – set out to prove the connection between the insect and the disease. It was an uphill task not only to do the difficult basic research work but to convince a skeptical military and medical establishment that their superstitious old theories of causation were of little use. The doctors even tried to use themselves as guinea pigs. Lazear went so far as to infect himself from a yellow-fever-carrying *Aedes* mosquito. This proved all too successful and it took him less than two weeks to die from the disease that he mistakenly believed he had developed immunity to.

But if the Commission proved the connection (although many others in the past had suggested it) it fell to Chief Sanitary Officer, William Gorgas (later to be of Panama Canal fame) to do something about it. Gorgas had virtually dictatorial power with a personality to match in occupied Havana at the turn of the 19th century. His soldiers roamed the city looking for any place the *Aedes* might breed; water pots and rain barrels were either emptied or smashed. Any person found with mosquito larvae on their property was heavily fined. Ponds were oiled every week. In just five months yellow fever was gone from the city.

Further north, New Jersey's chief entomologist John Smith launched a similar anti-mosquito campaign using a ditch-cutting machine designed for the purpose. His military-style 'mosquito brigades' covered the state, spraying oil on any waters that might act as breeding sites. Soon New Jersey beaches and other recreational areas that had been barely useable in mosquito season were popular once more.

Smith and Gorgas provide early models of what could be done on a local level using relatively low-tech methods to combat mosquito infestation. Such methods work well as a part of an overall public health approach that includes proper sanitation and screening. And despite the various agro-chemical and pharmaceutical innovations, this approach remains an anchor for keeping the mosquito at bay.

Fever trail

In the early days before the mosquito was identified as a disease source, and causation for malaria and other tropical fevers was a matter of (sometimes quite wild) speculation, the search for a cure was nonetheless pursued with great vigor. Back in the mid-1600s Spanish of all classes were suffering in the far reaches of the western Latin American region of their Empire. Then rumor associated with Jesuit missionaries who had spent time in the interior began to circulate about a special 'fever bark' that indigenous peoples used to provide relief for these illnesses. At that time, remember, malaria was

---

MALARIA MAP

There is no place on earth that is off the malaria map: Arctic Circle, freezing mountaintop, burning desert, you name it malaria's been there. We are not talking millions of cases here, more like hundreds of millions... And even when it's properly diagnosed, it's not like quinine is always going to get you home safe. With certain types of quinine, you can mainline malaria all the livelong day and come the nightfall you will still be gathering freezer-burn in the mortuary. ◆

Amitav Ghosh, *The Calcutta Chromosome*
(William Morrow, 1997).

---

not only a serious problem in tropical climates but also plagued Europe, particularly lowland Southern Europe. Once the word was out about the 'fever bark' a kind of mini-goldrush took place into the Amazon rainforest to find the red cinchona tree. The tree was actually the source of quinine which was to be the main source of relief from malaria for centuries to come.

The search for magic bark and the red cinchona (and other less productive trees) is well documented by Mark Honigsbaum in his lively history *The Fever Trail*. It is a fascinating story complete with fakes, frauds, dangerous expeditions and indigenous resistance to what came to be seen as bio-piracy particularly in places such as Bolivia.

Quinine and colonialism

There was a strong connection between quinine, colonialism and militarism. Malaria could have a devastating effect on army operations, putting entire battalions out of action. The death toll was frequently greater (often much greater) than that exacted by the foe. Indeed when the enemy was indigenous they may well have developed a level of immunity to keep them in much better fighting form.

This was the case right up through the World Wars of

the last century, and with quinine the main source of relief the scramble for control of supply was marked by much scheming and speculation. There were many attempts to transplant cinchona from its native Latin American habitat and the treacherous conditions for its extraction to more easily controlled plantations of the colonial empire. The history of manipulation of supply and price for quinine has an uncanny resemblance to the modern petroleum market. Eventually the wily Dutch merchant class working with Javanese planters in Indonesia grabbed a stranglehold on cinchona and the production of quinine. By the early 20th century, working through the Kina Bureau in Amsterdam, they had managed to seize control of 80 per cent of the world's supply.[4]

But the days of King Quinine were numbered. Once the source of disease was identified effort shifted to disease prevention through various strategies of mosquito abatement. Quinine-resistance also began to build in some of the pathogens. Artificial means of production were developed; newer and more effective substitutes were discovered. Other vaccines proved much more efficient as prophylactics. But today, quinine remains an affordable form of relief for hundreds of thousands of poor malaria sufferers.

3 Mosquitoes in uniform

'Mosquitoes are the fattest inhabitants
of this republic.'

FRED D'AGUIAR, GUYANAN WRITER

As is clear by now, there is an intimate relationship between the fate of armies and the ubiquitous mosquito. It is this that led historian CH Melville to pronounce: 'The history of malaria in war might almost be taken as the history of war itself.' We have seen how colonial armies with little or no immunity to malaria and yellow fever were often riddled with disease. This pattern held true right through the 20th century.

During World War One, British and French forces fighting near Salonika (Thessaloníki) in northern Greece were assaulted not by Germans but by malarial mosquitoes. In the summer of 1916 an Anglo-French Expeditionary Force landed to reinforce Serb allies in the Balkans. Unbeknownst to them this was not only the height of mosquito season but also thousands of Greek refugees infected with *falciparum* malaria were flooding into the area from Turkey. It made for a perfect storm of infection – a multitude of hungry mosquitoes with a ready source of infection to pass on.

The consequences were catastrophic. By the fall of the next year there were 30,000 cases amongst the troops. When a worried British commander called for French reinforcements for fear of being overrun by the Germans the response was cryptic but to the point: 'Regret that my army is in hospital with malaria.' The commander need not have worried as the German army was also reeling from the disease.[4]

From General MacArthur's forces in the South Pacific in World War Two to the US Operation Restore Hope in Somalia in the 1990s, the bite of the lowly mozzie was the main source of casualties.

Innovation on mosquito abatement and treatment strategies took a quantum leap forward during war. Quinine production was ramped up and research into new, more effective drugs took off. But this could be a two-edged sword as the legacy of the US war in Vietnam indicates. Malaria and mosquitoes were a huge problem in that conflict. US troops were dosed with drugs, first with chloroquine and when that proved ineffective they used mefloquine and halofantrine. Few soldiers actually died of malaria due to these ministrations. But in the urgency of war conditions, little attention was paid to the misuse of such drugs. So one of the legacies of the Vietnam débâcle is that malaria parasites developed a tolerance for all these drugs. Drug-resistant malaria crept across Asia and down into Africa.

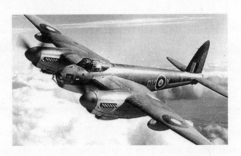

The Mosquito bomber

Another aspect of mosquitoes and warfare is quite different. It is the smallish bomber made by the de Havilland Company during World War Two, one of the most cost-effective aircraft ever built. The Mosquito was

MOZZIES AND DOODLEBUGS

From Edmonton, Alberta, Russ Bannock was Canada's second highest-scoring flying ace of World War Two. Born Russ Bahnuk in 1919, his father changed the family name to Bannock in 1939, as they were originally Austrian. His Germanic name was thought a problem at this period, especially as he had two cousins in the German Luftwaffe/air force. Growing up, Bannock did the usual prairie stuff, playing hockey and baseball. But he dreamt of becoming a pilot. In a 1989 interview he said: 'I grew up in Edmonton – always known for aviation in those days.'

He gained his pilot's license and in September 1939 when the War started, he became a Royal Canadian Air Force (RCAF) pilot. In 1943 he learned to fly the new Mosquito fighter/bomber and in June 1944 was sent to join 418 Squadron in England. Three days later the Germans started what is called the Second Battle of Britain, using their new V-1 unpiloted rockets. These were the *Vergeltungswaffen* or 'vengeance weapons'; also known as 'buzz-bombs' or 'doodlebugs' – the forerunners of today's Cruise Missiles.

The terror these new weapons caused was huge; each delivered 2,000 lbs of high explosive; they were aimed only

made of wood: Ecuadorian balsa for the plywood skin, Sitka spruce from Alaska and British Columbia in the wing spar, Douglas fir stringers, birch and ash for the longitudinal parts; all held together with glue and wood roughly at targets, so there was no knowing where or when they would fall. They had a pulse engine that made a putt-putt sound, until the fuel ran out and then they fell to earth to detonate.

The Mosquito was one of the few aircraft with the power to beat the buzz-bombs. 'Mozzies' went into the battle with instructions to intercept and destroy the doodlebugs over the English Channel if possible so that their explosion and fall wouldn't hurt anything.

Bannock developed tactics to combat the V-1s. Once a pilot spotted a bomb he had 30 seconds to plan and set up a shot. As soon as the rocket's highly flammable fuel erupted the pilot had to haul his plane rapidly away from the debris. Bannock's keen eyes and reflexes gave him a distinct edge. He decided the best way to stop V-1s was to catch them at their launch pads. On 3 July 1944 he headed for Abbeville, France, and saw a stream of V-1s starting to take off. Despite heavy flak his plane repeatedly attacked the site destroying many rockets.

He received the Distinguished Flying Cross, and later the Distinguished Service Order. He returned home to join De Havilland Canada as a sales director and test pilot. ◆

http://www.constable.ca/bannock.htm

screws. Its name probably came from its speed (faster than the famous and much lighter Spitfire) and power to 'sting'. With a crew of two the twin-engine Mosquito could carry the same bomb load to Berlin as the four-engine US

Flying Fortress with a crew of 11. It also did it a lot faster and used less fuel.

The 'Mozzie' was involved in high-profile raids over Germany. Hermann Goering, chief of the Luftwaffe, was outraged: 'The British, who can afford aluminum better than we can, knock together a beautiful wooden aircraft that every piano factory over there is building... There is nothing the British do not have. They have geniuses and we have the nincompoops. After the War's over I'm going to buy a British radio set – then at least I'll own something that has always worked.'[5]

The Mosquito ended up as the workhorse of the Royal Air Force who used it as a fighter-bomber, for photo-reconnaissance, trainer, torpedo-bomber, U-boat killer, mine-layer and target tug. It was the fastest bomber into the 1950s and remained in service into the 1960s.

4 Globalized mosquitoes

'The mosquito is more dangerous than the tiger.'

THAI PROVERB

The usual habitat of an individual mosquito is no more than a few miles (7 or 8 at most) from where they were hatched. It is within this territory that they reproduce, feed, take their blood meal if female and die. For tens of thousands of years before humans this was the case. Occasionally a mosquito will get caught in the winds and get blown hundreds of miles. Some have been found at altitudes way above 5,000 feet. But by and large their natural territory is small.

However we have played a big role in changing that by introducing new mosquito species into areas previously free of them. And with the mosquito can come pathogens that play havoc with human health.

An early example of how a mozzie can hitch a ride on modern transport is found in the Northeastern Brazilian port city of Natal, in 1930. A clutch of *Anopheles gambiae* stowed away on a fast French destroyer delivering mail from Africa. These mosquitoes are the most ferocious carriers of malaria. The hard-pressed local authorities in Rio Grande del Norte state ignored early warnings and suggestions that they flood recently-created local hayfields where the African mozzies were breeding. The results were catastrophic – starting with a local epidemic that sickened 10,000 people. Measures were belatedly taken and the mosquito was driven out of Natal but not out of the Northeast.

After a few local epidemics the *Anopheles* hit hard again in 1939, precipitating the largest malaria epidemic in the history of the Western hemisphere. Over 100,000 people fell sick with an estimated 20,000 getting a fatal dose. The local agricultural economy was devastated due to a lack of labor to either plant or harvest. It took a massive campaign of eradication including hit squads spraying indoor insecticides and outdoor larvaecides, drainage projects and roadblocks to spray outgoing traffic, trains, boats and planes. After months of work, over 4,000 Brazilian volunteers, under the command of an American, Fred Soper (who enjoyed virtually martial law powers), managed to drive the *Anopheles gambiae* out of Brazil saving the Americas from a malaria epidemic of unimaginable proportions.

Asian tigers

But the African *Anopheles* is not the only mosquito globetrotter. Take the ferocious Asian Tiger Mosquito, named for its stripes, size and voracious feeding and mating habits. The Tiger is a 'tree-hole mosquito' that breeds in water-filled cavities such as coconut husks or tree rot in her native Asia.

Enter the globalized trade in used tires. Recapping used tires for resale is illegal in Japan and Taiwan but not in the US and elsewhere. So each year millions of such tires are shipped to Houston, Texas – the tire recapping capital of the world. And guess who goes along for the ride. The water in these tires makes them perfect maternity wards for the Tigers. It was soon noticed by picnickers near the Houston Ship Channel that a new ferocious mosquito was destroying their previously pleasant pastime. From Houston the tires – and the mosquitoes – were shipped all over North America and to points South. With an

> **MOSQUITO FISH (*GAMBUSIA AFFINIS*)**
>
> Native to southern and eastern parts of the United States, mosquito fish can eat 100 to 500 larvae per day. They play an important role in mosquito control in ponds, canals, irrigated fields and some other freshwater sources. ◆

estimated four billion tires piled up all over the US, the breeding possibilities are almost endless.

Or take the *Aedes aegypti* that was responsible for the outbreak of dengue fever in Cuba in the 1970s. Cuba had previously been dengue-free and was pretty upset when its sugarcane crop started to rot in the fields because fever-stricken workers could not work. The Cubans accused the US Central Intelligence Agency of engineering the outbreak – not so outlandish a charge given the decades of US plotting against the Cuban revolution. Cuba launched a highly effective eradication campaign using authoritarian methods to eliminate the threat.

But soon the *Aedes aegypti* became a Latin America-wide issue as countries started to realize that this potential dengue-carrier was flourishing in the US ports of Galveston, Miami and New Orleans – the very ports from which goods were shipped to Latin America. Soon pressure was being applied through the Organization of American States for the US to clean up its act. But although the US had the vector mosquito they didn't have the pathogen (disease) to create a sense of urgency. When they did finally launch a control program it was tied up in the courts as US citizens resisted intrusion onto their property to get at the flying pests. The program was abandoned and while the *Aedes* has been controlled farther South it still flourishes in the US – much to the

AIDS

The HIV virus that produces AIDS in humans does not develop in mosquitoes. If HIV-infected blood is taken up by a mosquito, the virus is treated like food and digested along with the blood meal. If the mosquito takes a partial blood meal from an HIV-positive person and resumes feeding on a non-infected individual, insufficient particles are transferred to initiate a new infection.

If a fully engorged mosquito with HIV-positive blood is squashed on the skin, there would be insufficient transfer of virus to produce infection. The virus diseases that use insects as agents of transfer produce tremendously high levels of parasites in the blood. The levels of HIV that circulate in human blood are so low that HIV antibody is used as the primary diagnosis for infection. ◆

http://www.tlch2o.com/courses/MosquitoControl.pdf

consternation of Latin American health authorities who fear an outbreak of dengue, with imported US mosquitoes acting as vectors.

So mosquitoes as well as bankers and sweatshop-owners have benefited from globalization and the travel technologies on which it is based. And the same nation-states that scramble to control currency speculation and profit-repatriation are also scrambling to control infestations of alien mosquito species. Entire cargos and planes full of passengers are sprayed on arrival. Australia is particularly vigilant in this regard. Sometimes goods are put into quarantine or banned outright because of the risk. And local outbreaks of malaria known as 'airport malaria' have been identified near international airports.

5 Politics of prevention

'He can swallow a camel but chokes on a mosquito.'
LEBANESE PROVERB

As discussed earlier malaria, especially in its early period, was caught up with overt racism. Who got it? Who 'spread' it? Who got protected? All these questions were scarred by racism. This has changed in word if not in deed. There is concern for all sufferers of malaria but it has become cast, like many diseases, as a disease of poverty. While wealthy Northerners can and do still get sick it is essentially a disease of the developing countries. When Northern tourists, business people or aid workers go to malaria-infected areas they usually stay in healthy, screened locations. They dose themselves with a cocktail of prophylactic pharmaceuticals. But most of the 2.5 million people who are in the firing line of resurgent malaria are without these protections. Their poverty means they have neither the political clout to ensure that they have adequate public health systems or the market power to make it profitable for the international pharmaceutical cartel to invest what would be necessary to produce effective new products.

In the best of cases finding a 'cure' for malaria would be a Herculean task. Malaria's comeback has been marked by two kinds of resistance: that of the mosquito to the insecticide DDT and other chemical pesticides, and that of the malaria pathogen to historically effective quinine derivatives, and more recently to chloroquine and other modern treatments. One of the problems is that the malarial infectious agent is a very complex matter. This makes it different from other disease-causing microbes that are more amenable to treatment. Malaria parasites have up to 7,000 genes. These go through several development stages and a vaccine for one stage is useless at the next. And there is an almost endless variety of malaria parasites. If you develop a vaccine for one in a particular locality, then head a couple of hundred miles down the road, that same vaccine is useless.

Malaria (like cancer) is not one disease but a complex of diseases so no one vaccine is likely to work on all strains. This is compounded by parasites' capacity to develop resistance, rendering the once-successful fruitless. With no single drug entirely effective, developing a new anti-malarial is quite an expensive proposition. Health economists estimate that to produce results, at least half a billion dollars a year needs to be put into developing new anti-malarials.

Dragging their feet

With a few exceptions (such as the Swiss-based Novartis AG and its anti-malarial Coartem) the drug industry has shown very little interest. The current expenditure is less than $100 million a year. This is far less than is spent on cancer or other disease research and a mere $45 or less (depending on which mortality estimate you take) for each fatal case. Currently the more complex malaria parasite receives only a tenth of the funding going into AIDS research.

Between 1975 and 1999, only 4 of the 1,393 new drugs developed worldwide were anti-malarials. To get the big pharmaceutical corporations interested, Harvard economist Jeffery Sachs has proposed a publicly-supported vaccine purchase fund that would guarantee a market for effective anti-malarial vaccines and drugs. If implemented this could provide a billion-dollar market every year. But it's a big 'if'. As it stands Big Pharma continues to concentrate on finding cures for more profitable diseases despite some widely publicized pump-priming by wealthy philanthropists – such as Bill Gates who put $50 million into a Malaria Vaccine Initiative. This has been used to fund several promising vaccine candidates, the most hopeful of which is called RTS,S (sic) which has reportedly cut the rate of infection in Mozambican children aged one to four by 58 per cent. While important this is still a mere drop in the bucket. Even if a vaccine were developed it is not clear how it could be delivered to the most vulnerable populations around the world, particularly the young children of Africa.

Mugabe madness

There is another more localized and cruder form that the politics of prevention takes. In many countries around the world it is favored regions and groups that have the best access to anti-malarials and mosquito abatement programs. Sometimes this is a question of money, sometimes of political loyalties. Take the Mugabe regime in Zimbabwe. By the fall of 2005 Zimbabwe stood on the brink of a severe malaria epidemic. This despite the fact that major parts of southern Africa had witnessed decades of effective control of the *Anopheles* mosquito.

Richard Tren, director of Africa Fighting Malaria, laid the blame directly at Mugabe's feet: 'The problem is largely financial, and it seems Mugabe prefers to spend his money on shopping trips to Malaysia and on the Central Intelligence Organization than on public health.' And it's not just a question of budget priorities. The Mugabe regime has politicized its anti-malarial program, restricting individual treatment and preventive spraying to members of its ZANU-PF party. The regime's Operation Murambatsvina which drove hundreds of thousands of people (mostly opposition supporters) out of Harare and other centers and left them exposed to malaria in the countryside has played a big part in the resurgence of the disease. According to one report, 'We have witnessed many deaths of people who were evicted from urban areas. Malaria is even worse than HIV/AIDS. At least that disease gives you time to seek medication. But malaria kills very quickly. In some cases people have been denied medication and not allowed to buy food from shops because they are suspected of being MDC [opposition] supporters.'[6]

REMEMBER THE FLIT GUN?

'I wonder how many of us remember the flit gun – that large piece of domestic equipment the size of a garden spray and filled with a solution of DDT designed to deal with mozzies and other entomological intruders? Aimed in the wrong direction and filled with too strong a solution, the flit gun was capable of killing a pet budgie or acting like teargas on the assembled family. Then came Rachel Carson and *The Silent Spring*, and suddenly DDT disappeared. Perhaps most of us identify rather with the aerosol age – so much more compact and allegedly deadly – but, as we discovered to our cost as the ozone layer developed gigantic holes, driven by CFC-propellants which caused more deadly harm and on a wider scale to the greater environment. Each "advance" in the commercial application of "science" seemed to create more problems than it solved.'

From a speech by Professor Paul Walters, Rhodes University, South Africa.

While Zimbabwe provides a particularly heavy-handed example, the bias in treatment and prevention programs based on ethnic loyalty, political reliability or economic means is quite widespread. It is ironic that in Zimbabwe (as elsewhere) selective treatment undermines any overall prevention strategy. It is impossible to safeguard ZANU-PF members if their neighbors have the disease. Similarly the collapse of Zimbabwe's anti-malarial programs is bound to cross borders and affect neighboring countries.

The DDT controversy

DDT (*dichlorodiphenyl trichloroethane*) was first used in World War Two as a delousing agent. In 1948 the Swiss chemist Paul Müller was awarded the Nobel Prize for having discovered this extraordinary pesticide 9 years earlier. DDT was rapidly seen as a miracle cure for 'eradicating' mosquito-borne diseases. It had the same aura of magical technology about it as nuclear power does today for some people. The late 1950s and early 1960s was an era of endless technological optimism. The campaign to wipe out malaria and eliminate mosquitoes as a species was tied up with the Cold War attempt by the US to present itself as the alternative to communism. The DDT-based campaign spearheaded by USAID (overseas aid) and the Rockefeller Foundation was meant to be the human face of the US Empire. DDT factories sprang up around the world. Spraying took place both indoors and outdoors.

It is undeniable that DDT saved millions of lives. Malaria was wiped out in islands including Taiwan, Sardinia and Jamaica. Rates of infection plummeted in

Sri Lanka and India. By 1961 malaria had been eliminated or dramatically reduced in 37 countries.

But then doubts began to emerge. Evidence grew that DDT is what is called a 'bio-accumulator'. The higher up the food chain you got the more this persistent organic pollutant (POP) was found in the tissues of fish and mammals. In 1962 Rachel Carson's ecological classic *The Silent Spring* rang alarm bells about a future without birdsong. The reproduction process of everything from eagles to humans was impacted. Hormone-disruption was seen to cause premature human births and 'black holes' – areas where certain species of wildlife disappeared almost entirely. Today DDT residues are part of a larger chemical stew of POPs with unsure but frightening implications. Evidence of collateral damage in the fight against the lowly mosquito started to create some serious misgivings.

Battle lines

So the stage was set for a battle between those – often besieged health authorities in poor countries – who held onto DDT as a matter of immediate life-or-death and those concerned with the long-term (and not so long-term) environmental implications of over-reliance on DDT. There was also a group of media-savvy pro-corporate (mostly US) hucksters who denied any negative impact of DDT at all and denounced all such findings as 'junk science' put out by self-serving environmentalists. Such people, as with those who deny all climate change, are outside the bounds of reasonable debate. Their motivations are more ideological and pecuniary.

There is however a legitimate debate between those who feel there is no place for DDT and those who think that the human toll of mosquito-borne diseases weighs heavier in the balance than more diffuse environmental effects. The website of the World Health Organization (WHO) mirrors some of the schizophrenia involved with strong statements encouraging both the continued use and the phasing out of DDT.

In 1999 South Africa experienced the worst outbreak of malaria it has seen in decades with almost 61,000 cases. The Government resorted to previously curtailed indoor spraying of DDT and the rates of infection fell dramatically.

It seems unlikely that DDT will be phased out entirely, especially during epidemics of mosquito-borne diseases in poor sub-Saharan African countries. However it has become quite clear that the chemical is not the miracle cure it was once thought to be.

There is an increasing problem with DDT-resistant mosquitoes. These were first identified in India in 1959 and have the capacity to increase dramatically as part of the overall mosquito population as non-resistant mosquitoes are wiped out. It takes about five years for a mosquito population to develop a complete resistance to DDT. That is the window of opportunity to dry up a reservoir of pathogens in a human population.

A more holistic approach to mosquito control involves the utilization of bednets and other prophylactic devices, the reduction of mosquito-breeding habitats, the selective use of pesticides, overall public health improvement of infrastructure and through education, the slowing of drug resistance and environmental decisions that do not increase human exposure.

Some DDT use has nothing to do with mosquito-control and is simply an excuse to continue spraying it as a cheap agricultural pesticide.[7]

In 1969 WHO declared an end to their campaign of species elimination against the mosquito as a way of getting rid of malaria. It has been replaced by a more modest campaign to 'Roll Back Malaria'. Their admitted failure was a failure of their main weapon: DDT. So DDT is at best a monocultural (and thus partial) solution to what is a diverse and very tricky problem. If we are going to outsmart the wily mosquito we will have to do better than that.

Malaria resurgence

You can see the pattern from Sri Lanka to Guyana. The malaria vector is driven out by heavy DDT spraying in combination with other means. The instance of malaria drops dramatically almost to the point of extinction. A few years pass and the mosquitoes come back tougher than ever and not deterred by a few agro-chemicals. Local people have lost the partial immunity they once had to various strains of malaria. Instant healthcare crisis.

With the growth of DDT and drug/vaccine resistance, malaria is storming back. Gone is all talk of malaria eradication and the elimination of the mosquito as its vector. From 1970 to 1997, global mortality rates for the disease increased by 13 per cent. Death rates in sub-Saharan Africa jumped by 54 per cent in the same period. Malaria-specific deaths among African children have leapt by nearly one-third since the 1960s, wiping out gains made against a clutch of other childhood diseases.

Add to this the spread of other mosquito-borne diseases such as West Nile virus and Rift Valley fever and the notion of a science-based eradication looks distinctly shaky. Then there is the question of climate instability that opens up mosquito opportunities through changes in rainfall patterns and a rise in temperatures.

Environmental disruption

Human manipulation of the environment changes the habitat for mosquitoes as it does for all other species. Sometimes breeding areas such as swamps are wiped out and the mosquito (or some types) decline. Urban water is often too polluted to support mosquito breeding. But the interaction between mosquitoes and different parts of the environment is extraordinarily complex. For example an increase in livestock population can reduce the tendency to take blood from people. But mechanization of agriculture could cause mosquitoes that used to get their blood from livestock to switch to people. This happened in the late 1960s when malaria returned to Guyana after the *Anopheles aquasalis* changed its habits to adapt to the lack of livestock, its preferred source for a blood meal.

Deforestation can also enhance conditions. Between 1974 and 1991 Brazil witnessed a ten-fold increase in malaria due mostly to logging in the Amazon. The vector *Anopheles Darlingi* thrived on the sunnier forest edge instead of the deep rainforest. Irrigation schemes and dam-building can also increase exposure by providing new attractive breeding areas. The large Mahawehli River Project in Sri Lanka created more land under cultivation but also brought malaria back into areas from which it had been eradicated. Mega-projects are fraught with potential problems, but this does not have to be so. The Tennessee Valley Authority which built a whole dam system in the US during the 1930s Depression consciously 'designed out' mosquito habitat by use of artificial canals, angled slopes and frequent changes in water level. These efforts were widely recognized as helping drive malaria out of the US South.

As we have seen, micro-environment is also crucial. Mud-brick construction leaves holes in the ground which are perfect breeding sites, and we already know about water containers...

And so they get everywhere, biting and buzzing, annoying us: 'The mosquito is without a soul, but its whizzing vexes the soul,' goes a Turkish saying. But even so, we let them in to our music, art and culture as seen in the next chapter.

6

Mosquito culture

'He felt like a drunken giant walking with the
limbs of a mosquito'
THINGS FALL APART BY CHINUA ACHEBE

**The mosquito evokes the evasive, the sneaky,
the** determined, the swarming, the multitude, the
unstoppable. In cartoons mozzies are sometimes
portrayed as tall and sinister. They can be the stuff of
doom, but on a more positive note they can represent the
'small but tough'. It can be an image of terror but also one
of humor and fun. The mosquito has inspired everything
from the titles of novels to the younger divisions of little
league baseball. There is Paul Theroux's *Mosquito Coast*

(named after a region in Central America) and William Faulkner's 1927 novel *Mosquito*. There's a modernist novel by Dan Jones (*Mosquito*) and a stack of children's literature.

And there is even poetry in mosquitoes if you look for it. Here's a fragment from DH Lawrence's elegant poem *The Mosquito*:

What do you stand on such high legs for?
How can you put so much devilry
Into that translucent phantom shred
Of a frail corpus?

There is a book of poetry by the Japanese-American poet Kimiko Hahn (*Mosquito and Ant*). Hahn wrote: 'I want my letters to imitate mosquitoes as they loop around the earlobe... the impossible task of slapping one....'

Perhaps the most intriguing work is a thriller by VA MacAllister (*The Mosquito War*) about a frustrated Vietnamese lab assistant, whose mother and brother died of malaria, and who is driven to bio-terrorism. He tosses two jarfuls of mosquitoes bearing a fatal strain of malaria into a crowd of shoppers in a Washington mall on Independence Day. It's got everything including corporate bigwigs at a Big Pharma company cutting funding for a potential malaria cure.

African writers such as Chinua Achebe not surprisingly mention mosquitoes in their literature. In his famous work *Things Fall Apart*, Achebe tells the story of the mosquito, one of several West African tales which explain why these insects buzz irritatingly in people's ears:

'Okonkwo... woke up in the middle of the night. He scratched his thigh where a mosquito had bitten him as he slept. Another one was wailing near his right ear. He slapped his ear and hoped he had killed it. Why do they always go for one's ears?

When he was a child his mother had told him a

WHAT'S IN A NAME?

The Miskito ethnic group in Central America was formed when black slaves ran away to live in La Mosquitia rainforest and intermarried with local Indians. The area is famous as the setting for Paul Theroux's novel *The Mosquito Coast*.

The origin of the Miskito name is not the Mosquito. Some say their name comes from the British musket that they used to use, but the Miskitos themselves say they are descended from a group of people who followed a chief called Miskut. Today, they are active in protecting their rainforest, bilingual education (Miskito-Spanish), and for the development of Mosquitia with schools and clinics. ◆

story about it... Mosquito had asked Ear to marry him, whereupon Ear fell on the floor in uncontrollable laughter. "How much longer do you think you will live?" she asked. "You are already a skeleton." Mosquito went away, humiliated, and any time he passed her way he told Ear that he was still alive.'

There are festivals, like the annual Great Texas Mosquito Festival where you can hear some excellent country music. This Festival even has its own massive yellow mosquito mascot, and also an event named the Mosquito Calling Contest: 'Those pesky mosquitoes are buzzing around ready to be called into the park by that special sound, call, or voice. You will not want to miss out on this one-of-a-kind event. So mark your calendar and don't forget to bring your cheering squad to share in the excitement of the moment. Remember, it is open season for those pros that can call the largest, fastest, and bloodsucking mosquito around.'

If Texas isn't in your plans you could hit the mosquito festival in the little town of Paisley, Oregon. Or then if you prefer Canada, there is a mozzie festival in Fort-Coulonge on the Ottawa River.

There are computer games like Mister Mosquito or Mosquito Blaster. Then there are a range of other games

MOSQUITOES GET EVERYWHERE...

Big Game Hunting

Some hunters talking together; each says that he is packing a heavier and more powerful gun to shoot with. The first starts out with a small handgun and the last ending up with a very powerful rifle, shotgun, whatever.

Two others come over who have overheard the hunters and want to settle a bet. Are the hunters going after wolves or moose? One of the hunters replies, 'Why no, we are going after mosquitoes!' ◆

The MacScouter's Big Book of Skits, R Gary Hendra.
www.macscouter.com

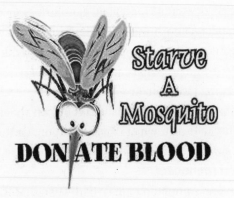

that can have you swatting virtual mosquitoes on your computer all day long. While the mosquito doesn't exactly lend itself to use on coins and stamps the way, say, a lion or eagle does, it is still there, often looking quite ominous, on postage stamps from Mexico to Haiti and the old USSR. Most of these images are in use to either commemorate or encourage some anti-malarial campaign or other.

Mozzies have been around a very long time – perhaps as long as 25 million years; certainly there are some ancient specimens caught and preserved in amber (tree sap). You can buy one, which the ad from the supplier in the Dominican Republic emphasizes is 'very uncommon' and centuries old. Yours for a mere $525. Add it to your collection of prehistoric spiders and grasshoppers trapped in amber.

But if that's a little much perhaps you might like the nifty little Sig Sauer Mosquito – a handgun. The folks at Sauer and Sohn promise 'a thousand rounds without a stiff arm and a hole in your wallet! Sound good? No problem with the MOSQUITO.' The tough and small imagery lends itself particularly well to the marketing of handguns.

Guns and teenagers

Or maybe you are being annoyed by the one thing that some people find worse than mosquitoes – teenagers.

Well, Bill Stapleton, a security consultant and inventor from Wales has just the solution. He has produced a 'small and annoying' device called the Mosquito that emits a high-pitched noise that almost no-one over 30 and everyone under 20 can hear. Stapleton, who road-tested his invention on his own children, claims that a convenience store that installed the device had troublesome teenagers begging the storeowner to 'turn it off'. More recently the mosquito Trojan computer virus (notice how sneaky they are!) is currently infecting smart

MEET MISTER MOSQUITO

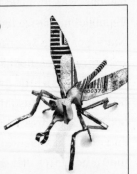

Mister Mosquito is a video game for PlayStation 2. You play as a comical cartoon mosquito ('Mr Moskeeto') and you must stock up on blood through the summer so that you may survive the winter ahead. To do this Mr Moskeeto has taken up residence in the house of the Yamada family: father Kenichi, mother Kaneya and teenage daughter Rena. Kenichi enjoys flower arranging while wife Kaneya is a hobby photographer, Rena is a student about to go on a trip who listens to Progressive Jazz and is into martial arts. ◆

Wikipedia

phones when downloaded as part of a popular mosquito computer game.

Mosquito obsession

In the logging and mining camps of Northern Canada where the pay is good and workers often pass months on end, there is an obsession even greater than sex: the mosquito. If you are working outdoors and living in basic accommodation, they are your constant companions. You hate them! And the home remedies for keeping them at bay are endless. Some have to do with the kinds of clothes you wear. Never wear blue, looks too much like water where the pesky critters came from and where they feel at home. Best avoid dark entirely and wear bright clothes. This is also useful if you don't want to get shot by a wayward hunter! Then there is the smudge that has you choking on smoke for hours on end because the mozzies have the good sense not to.

A lot of the remedies have to do with smell – the more the better. For a start never wash. Then there are the concoctions often with bear grease as a base. Like I said, obsession. There is even a radio station in Northern Quebec which claims to emit a high-pitched sound beyond human hearing that drives mosquitoes away. Great for the ratings.

Zapping the buggers

A whole industry has grown up to keep mosquitoes away. Ironically it peddles its wares mostly to those for whom the buzzers are mostly a nuisance rather than a fatal peril. The trusty fly-swatter just ain't hi-tech enough. Rather try the effective chemical DEET, but don't overuse it because it can cause nerve damage. Then there is citronella but you've got to keep applying the damn stuff to keep them from crawling up your pant leg or under your

ALL THE THINGS A MOSQUITO CAN BE

A PLANT: Mosquito Fern or Azolla is a floating fern, colored from green to red and generally found in ponds protected from wind. They can be aggressive invaders and are often mixed in with duckweeds or watermeal. If these fern colonies cover the water, then oxygen depletion and fish kills can occur. Colonies of mosquito fern provide habitats for many micro and macro invertebrates which feed fish and other wildlife.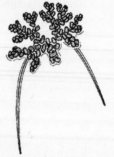

A RADIO AMPLIFIER: the Buzquito (or Mosquito) Amplifier http://sgauge.free.fr/mosquito/shema.jpg

A TORPEDO BOAT: HMQS Mosquito, Colonial Navy of Queensland Australia, launched in 1884 in England.

skirt. You could try 'Buzz Off' insect-repellant clothing. These days shelves are overflowing with sprays and coils, nets, liquids and lotions to take away the itch, electronic gizmos known hopefully as 'zappers' to electrocute the little buggers and take the sting out of the bite. There are even large versions of these outside pubs and bars so the patrons can enjoy an outdoor smoke. It's a million dollar growth industry. And what with global warming, maybe 'an emerging market' too.

A LEGO CONSTRUCTION:
'The Mosquito *small single-seat scout spacefighter* is an extremely compact scout. Its armament consists of two heavy cannons that can put up a good fight against other small fighters but are not effective on bigger craft. The Mosquito relies on its fast engine to speedily fly away from unwanted confrontations. Its cockpit can hold one pilot with little room to spare.'
ART: such as *Mosquito Bite* by AnneKarin Glass www.annekaringlass.com
A 'FLY' for fishing
A HANG-GLIDER in Argentina www.vuelomaximo.com.ar/
A BAND: 'Mosquito plays kick-ass rock with a lot of crazy vocals and electronic effects. They play with a variety of styles and are a very promising up and coming band in the Tokyo indie scene. Check them out!' www.yesjapan.com/mosquito/ ◆

BITING HUMOR

'DON'T FORGET YOUR PROTECTIVE ATTIRE IN INDIA'

It's oppressively hot in India, but you wouldn't know it from the way people dress. They wear saris, *salwar kameezes*, *kurtas* or other long garments; traditional clothing that was designed many years ago by people living in the North Pole. Some of those people migrated to India, but despite the stifling heat, decided not to change their clothing and expose more of their skin. They were concerned about morality, of course, but not as much as they were concerned about mosquitoes.

India isn't full of mosquitoes, but it has more than its fair share. That's why government officials, noticing the scarcity of mosquitoes in some countries, have wisely formed the Indian Mosquito Export Agency. If you live in a country that isn't blessed with mosquitoes, you can finally do something about it! Act now while supplies are high and prices are low!

There are many reasons to import mosquitoes. You can conduct research on them. You can keep them as pets. You can give them to friends at Christmas. Just remember this: Unlike cats, mosquitoes will not ignore you. You'll enjoy their company day and night.

Your investment is guaranteed to increase exponentially. Yes, buy 6 mosquitoes today and you'll have 200 in a few weeks. You can start your own mosquito supply company.

Don't worry about depleting India's mosquito resources. Thanks to good planning by the Government, India has built a large reserve of mosquitoes, enough to keep the world well-supplied for years. The country has so many mosquitoes that anyone who goes days without being bitten will eventually have this uneasy thought: 'What's wrong with my blood? Even the mosquitoes don't want it. Perhaps I should get it tested.'

If you're a musician performing in India, don't assume that the audience is clapping for you. They're probably swatting mosquitoes. In fact, many Indian classical dances have incorporated mosquito swatting into their movements. That gentle touch of the belly may seem subtle, but not to a mosquito.

Indians have learned to protect themselves from mosquitoes. Some sleep under nets, others cover their bodies with ointment, and a few try to repulse the buzzing pests by not taking baths. Perhaps the best protection is the Secured Attire for Resisting Insects (SARI). Mosquitoes aren't fond of saris, because each sari consists of yards of material that go around a woman's body. How many yards? Enough to wrap a dozen Egyptian mummies. In fact, the first 'mummy' was an Indian mummy who was laid to rest in her sari. The sari would be completely impenetrable if women weren't inclined to compromise function with style and allow a section of their stomachs to be visible. This is the section that attracts not just hordes of mosquitoes but also hordes of men.

A *salwar kameez* solves this problem quite nicely. For many women, it's the next best thing to wearing a suit of armor. They're well-protected from top to bottom, with plenty of overlap between the upper dress and lower pajama. The message to men and mosquitoes is clear: 'Don't even think about it.' ◆

Melvin Durai, Manitoba-based writer and humorist. A native of India, he grew up in Zambia. www.melvindurai.com

Some pretty weird contraptions have hit the stores – like the fogger/mist sprayer for temporary relief from flying mosquitoes. For that extra kick add 5 per cent malathion chemical to your fog; trouble is, malathion can cause cancer, and it hangs around for a long time. Then there are a variety of mosquito traps such as the New Jersey Light Trap or the Insect Electrocuter Light. Down on Key Island off Florida they claim to have developed a trap with bait of carbon dioxide and liquid octenol that (apparently) smells like cow's breath. This supposedly irresistible combination for salt marsh mosquitoes has reduced the pesky devils by 90 per cent in three years. No electric grid or pesticide involved. Hell, it's almost New Age 'appropriate technology' killing.

So why are we so obsessed with the lowly mosquito? Obviously in many places in the world it's a question of life and death. But the obsession seems greatest where the threat is mostly not that grave – or at least, not yet. Is it simply that we are genetically hardwired to a memory of centuries ago when the mosquito meant death from yellow fever? But that couldn't be, because back then we didn't know where the disease was coming from.

But today mozzies could be carrying West Nile virus or some weird bird flu that will start a pandemic. Maybe it's all those horror movies, like the ones about the giant ants attacking Los Angeles with James Arness starring as the head cop. Surely there had to be one about mosquitoes. Or maybe it's all about disposable income.

While all these are partially true, there is something else about the mosquito. They've been around since before the time of the dinosaurs. Their continued aggressive existence seems a slight to our mastery of nature. How dare they?

7 The future

'In heaven you won't hear the mosquitoes.'

FINNISH SAYING

Despite the loud protestations of oil-industry-funded skeptics it is now quite clear that our world is getting hotter: climate change is happening. A growing scientific consensus makes this crystal clear. And warmer temperatures broaden the range of disease-carrying mosquitoes. After years of decline malaria is on the increase with at least some locally-transmitted cases coming to light in places like New York State.

Then there are new kinds of mosquito-borne diseases such as West Nile virus that are currently taking their toll throughout North America. The UK's chief medical officer warned in 2001 that with a rise of a few degrees of temperature the local *Anopheles atroparvus* might change its nesting habits, and if a couple of feverish backpackers returning from Asia get bitten and... ? The implication: malarial hell could break loose in those tidy little English villages.

But the most immediate effects will be in Africa where mosquitoes have been found breeding in Kenya and elsewhere at 1,600 meters for the first time. The highlands of Africa were always a sanctuary from many mosquito-borne diseases, but climate change is calling that into question. Flooding that accompanies changes in rainfall patterns has already resulted in localized epidemics in Mozambique and the northern highlands of Burundi. Add to this collapsing public health systems (sacrificed on the altar of debt repayment) and mosquitoes developing a resistance to agrochemicals like DDT but also to strains of *falciparum malaria* that no longer respond to chloroquine or quinine.

Chinese medicine

Now the World Health Organization is warning against the misuse of *artemisinin* – a drug extracted from the dry leaves of a Chinese herb once thought to be the perfect mono-therapy for malaria. It was developed in Chinese laboratories suspicious of the motives and methods of Western Big Pharma. However, there is a catch: it turns out that if the full course of treatment (five days) is not taken, the parasite mutates and becomes resistant. The WHO is so concerned that it has called for an end to production of artemisinin except in combination with other drugs. But with a huge black market in both genuine and fake malaria cures this may be impossible to enforce. The 'battle' against the mosquito looks like anything but 'won'.

Way back in 1996 the Worldwatch Institute issued a disturbing paper which foresaw some of what is now coming to pass. It identified a pattern of exploding populations, rampant poverty, inadequate healthcare, misuse of antibiotics and severe environmental degradation that underlay a dramatic increase in infectious diseases. The report concluded that 'water pollution, shrinking forests and rising temperatures are driving the upward surge in infections in many countries. Beyond the number of people who die, the social and economic cost of infectious diseases is hard to overestimate. It can be a crushing burden for families, communities or governments.'

In Africa alone it is estimated that malaria over the last 35 years has led to a loss of $100 billion to the African economy – more than four times what the continent receives in international aid every year. The Worldwatch report concludes that 'the dramatic resurgence of infectious diseases is telling us that we are approaching disease and medicine, as well as economic development, the wrong way. Governments focus too narrowly on individual cures and not mass prevention.'[8] Climate change and its potential for increasing the range of pathogen-carrying mosquitoes is one good example of the limits of a narrow approach. Some estimates have it that, by 2050 malaria will return to the southern US, southern Brazil, western China and regions across central Asia. A holistic philosophy and policy that would prioritize public health gives us a chance, perhaps not to 'eradicate' the mosquito, but at least to put it in its place.

Search for the Magic Bullet

DDT, despite its undoubted uses, has proved not quite the solution that people thought it might be. Similarly a number of promising drugs have turned out to be of limited value. Both mosquitoes and the pathogens they carry have proved to have a resilient 'bounce back' capacity that defeats scientific researchers – at least in the long run. Still, faith in science is strong and the effort to find a single techno-solution is not easily discouraged. There are several high-tech possibilities, including a system of satellite mapping technology of anticipating outbreaks of malaria by tracking rainfall patterns.

Glow-in-the-dark testicles

Most of the attention (and a good deal of resources) in the search for a new magic bullet is being invested in genetic manipulation. The idea is to create a genetically-modified mosquito that cannot carry the malaria pathogen and then release it into the wild where it will breed with other mosquitoes, passing on its anti-malarial genes. The new mosquito will be 'vector impotent'. In order to separate out the males for release the clever scientists at the Imperial College in London have even added a gene that makes the mosquitoes' testicles fluorescent – they really do glow in the dark.

But Andrew Spielman, who has spent a good deal of his life trying to figure out and contain mosquitoes, is distinctly skeptical. He is convinced that there will be success in the lab but is dubious that this beautiful science can be translated into real world conditions. He is doubtful that lab mosquitoes can survive and compete for mates. He is wary that they may become vectors for new pathogens or mutated versions of old ones. He is also worried that people may accept these new 'beneficial' mosquitoes and give up their bednets and pesticides, thus allowing the pests to thrive. In his fascinating study *Mosquito* he concludes: 'In the countries, cities and villages in which malaria and the *Anopheles* do their damage, this approach will fail. The realities of both nature and humankind conspire, in many ways, to defeat the kinds of interventions planned by molecular biologists.'[2]

Another scientist, Robert S Desowitz, whose book *The Malaria Capers* exposed corruption and waste in the search for a cure-all vaccine, reached much the same conclusion back in the early 1990s. 'Expertise has been lost; the last generation of truly experienced "field hands" is leaving the scene, lost to age and disuse. They are being replaced by..."molecular types" more concerned with the exquisite intellectual challenges of modish science than with seeking practical solutions. The razzle-dazzle and promise of biotechnology have led Third World health officials to expect a quick fix – the malaria vaccine "just around the corner" or the genetically-altered mosquito... the last word in controlling vector-borne diseases.'[3]

What works

It all depends how you define success. As should be obvious by now, nothing is THE ANSWER. Some things work at least work partially. A lot of stock these days is being put in what is cheap and simple – the opposite of the expensive techno-fix. The bednet is a good example. Bednets are mosquito netting that is treated with a pyrethroid insecticide and then suspended over a bed or hammock. Occasionally the nets have to be re-treated with an insecticide to maintain their potency. Most *Anopheles* feed in the evening and at night so the nets can dramatically reduce the number of infective bites. Children who sleep under nets have shown declines in malaria of 14 to 63 per cent, with premature deaths dropping by 25 per cent.

Simple solutions

Nets are becoming increasingly popular, particularly in West African countries such as Senegal, Burkina Faso and Chad where they are almost standard in some areas. In the Gambia up to 80 per cent of the people now use nets. In rural Tanzania between 1997 and 1999 there was a 6-fold increase in net ownership and a 27 per cent increase in survival rates for children who sleep under them. Despite the positive Tanzanian results, nets have been less widely adopted in other places. Part of the reason for this is that many people do not sleep on beds, but on the floor and that makes using a net very difficult. There is also the cost, which has been aggravated by the fact that many African countries impose a tariff on their import thus forcing up the price. This has been widely condemned as a 'malaria tax' and governments have agreed to stop although most have not done so. Bednets remain a viable way of cutting malaria death rates, but it is likely that, if they are ever really going to catch on, they must be publicly underwritten. Most African villagers simply can't afford them. Public subsidy makes sound economic sense. After all, the $4 it would cost to supply each child with a bednet would be made up many times over by the reduction of losses to African economies from malaria.

Micro-managing the local environment can also reduce the threat from mosquitoes. If close attention is paid to reducing the possibility of breeding in or near human communities this will reduce the level of bites and infection. This is so because mosquitoes have a limited range. If stagnant or still water is nearby it should be closely monitored for larvae. One problem in Africa is that mud-bricks are used as building material particularly in rural areas. This usually involves digging up earth (and creating holes) near building sites to avoid having to carry the bricks long distances. These holes fill with water and provide a deluxe breeding place for mozzies. A combination of popular education and new building methods could help reduce infections.

In Vietnam a tiny freshwater copepod crustacean has been used to eliminate mosquito larvae from the water (and thus cut back dramatically on the mosquito population)

MAPPING MALARIA'S GENETIC CODE

New ways of tackling malaria are likely to be developed as a result of a new scientific milestone. A hundred years after the discovery that mosquitoes transmit the malaria parasite, the complete genetic codes of both the human malaria parasite and the mosquito that spreads it have been deciphered by an international team.

'It will be a little while before the knowledge provided by the genome projects is translated into practical tools but this will happen and malaria will finally be brought under control,' commented Professor Brian Greenwood, from the London School of Hygiene and Tropical Medicine, UK. 'The first mosquito resistant to the malaria parasite could be developed within a year,' he added.

But some researchers are skeptical about how quickly

in 37 rural communes. Finding and strategically placing the little larvae-eaters can be done by local people.

So a multi-pronged approach that includes insecticides and both science-intensive prophylactic and treatment drugs (hopefully some new ones) but also bednets and locally appropriate vector control appears the way to go. But mosquito-borne diseases should not be considered in isolation. It is a very hard-won lesson that so many of the indicators of marginalization in the Global

developments will happen in the new post-genomic era. They think funds would be better spent on vaccines and drugs that are already in the pipeline.

'If there were an extra £100m to spend on malaria-vaccine research, I would allocate very little of it to exploring the parasite genome,' said Professor Adrian Hill of Oxford University, UK, in the journal *Nature*.

And his caution was echoed by Chris Curtis, Professor of Medical Entomology at the London School of Hygiene and Tropical Medicine. He said: 'I'm skeptical that the *Anopheles* mosquito genome will actually be useful in attempts to control malaria in very poor countries and I have a feeling that projects on the genome are done because molecular biologists think they can be done and are exciting to do.' ◆

news.bbc.co.uk

South – population, crime, malnutrition, lack of rights and freedoms – are tangled up in the web of debt and exploitation in which such societies are caught. This is also true of modern disease, including persistent malaria. Economic security and a modest level of prosperity would make a huge difference to rates of infection and mortality. The public health care system all over the Global South is being sucked dry of funds in this era of neo-liberalism that emphasizes private provision and 'cost recovery' over the health of poor people. Decent housing, safe water and sanitation infrastructure would not only reduce infection but improve general health and immune-system resistance once infection does occur. Malaria and yellow fever are no longer serious problems in the industrial world (at least for the moment) largely because there is a minimum level of prosperity and public sanitation. Such advances would yield similar results elsewhere.

Conclusion

Even the most ardent deep ecologist will tell you it is hard to actually love (or even like) mosquitoes. Unlike the Panda Bear or Whooping Crane, which at least some of humankind is actually trying to save from extinction, it is quite likely we would wipe out the mosquito if we could.

But the fact is that we can't. And the fact that we can't says something about our relationship with nature. Maybe conquest isn't the way to go.

We may never learn to love the mosquito but perhaps we

NATURAL FOE?

Toxorhynchites, also known as mosquito hawk, is the only species of mosquito that does not suck blood. Rather, it preys on the larvae of other mosquitoes. The larvae of one jungle variety, the *Toxorhynchites splendens*, consume larvae of other mosquito species, particularly the *Aedes aegypti*. These cannibalistic mosquitoes are bigger in size but they do not attack people because they are not blood-suckers. The adult *Toxorhynchites splendens* subsists on nectar and other natural carbohydrates. Zairi Jaal, Vector Control Research Unit co-ordinator at Universiti Sains Malaysia, explains that as the *Toxorhynchites splendens* is a natural predator of *Aedes* larvae, it would be a suitable agent to help fight the menace of dengue. 'The mosquito will not bite humans and will not transmit any disease. We can breed the larvae and introduce them into tree holes or bring in adult mosquitoes for them to reproduce.' There are dozens of species of *Toxorhynchites* around the world and they share a similar trait – their larvae have a voracious appetite for the young of other mosquitoes. ◆

Wikipedia en.wikipedia.org

---

should learn to respect their ability to adapt and survive. After all they were here long before we were and odds are they may have more staying power as a species than we do. A little admiration might also be called for as our own adaptive skills could use a little honing. Mozzies have pretty much bounced back from all the human schemes to wipe them out. So like it or not we have to share the planet with them.

The mosquito has defeated our efforts because those efforts were (despite the application of our best science) far too simple-minded. We have tried again and again to find a single 'magic bullet' solution to deal with a complicated problem. We are still seeking such solutions – this time genetic rather than agro-chemical or pharmaceutical. It is likely that some of the resources would be of more use in the field than in the lab.

However, once we accept that we cannot conquer the mosquito but must live with it, we need to adopt a varied strategy that starts with knowledge (often quite local knowledge) about the pest and its reproduction strategy. We need to begin perhaps with that age-old adage – know your enemy. If we combine the undoubted advances of science with an on-the-ground knowledge about the habits of both people and mosquitoes we just might be able to do what the World Health Organization is now proposing and 'Roll Back Malaria'.

Perhaps we can learn from the mozzie's tactics, especially if we think we cannot do anything to change the world. Consider this: 'If you think you are too small to be effective, you have never been in bed with a mosquito.'

1 'A high-tech mosquito barrier', Shane Adams, *Agricultural Research*, March 1996. 2 Andrew Spielman and Michael D'Antonio, *Mosquito* (Hyperion, 2001). 3 Robert S Desowitz, *The Malaria Capers* (WW Norton, 1991). 4 Mark Honigsbaum, *The Fever Trail* (Macmillan, 2001). 5 A Short History of the DH98 Mosquito, www.home.gil.com. au 6 'Zimbabwe's cavalry', *The Zimbabwean*, 2 September, 2005. 7 'Combating Malaria', Anne Platt McGinn, *State of the World Report 2003*, UNICEF. 8 www.worldwatch.org/pubs/paper/129/

CONTACTS & RESOURCES

Websites

www.mosquito-zapper.com – an exhaustive source of information about the pesky mosquito.
www.whyfiles.org – more of the same.
www.newscientist.com – for the latest in scientific innovation in the great mosquito war.
www.bbc.co.uk – look up the edited guide entry 'Why Mosquitoes Must Die.'
www.cdc.gov – a US Government site on different types of disease.
www.melvindurai.com Melvin Durai is a Manitoba-based writer and humorist. A native of India, he grew up in Zambia.

Organizations

World Heath Organization – co-ordinates the 'Roll Back Malaria' campaign; great source of information about mosquito-borne diseases. www.who.int/eng
The People's Health Movement – an international forum of health activists and networks from around the world, mixing concern for public health with that of social justice. www.phmovement.org – good source of contacts for activist groups and networks.

HealthWrights – a non-profit organization committed to advancing the health, basic rights, social equality, and self-determination of disadvantaged persons and groups. www.healthwrights.org
Global Health Watch – South African-based organization which is 'a call to all health workers to broaden and strengthen the global community of health advocates.' www.ghwatch.org